PRO BODY BUILDING TIPS,
The complete guide to bodybuilding training for men

Cent OZ

Table of contents

chapter 1

The Complete Guide to Bodybuilding: All the Information You Need

Want to gain weight like you're getting paid to? This is how.

Five Tips from a Pro Bodybuilder for Building Muscle

The majority of people believe bodybuilders to be "mass monsters" and often unhealthily-appearing individuals, says Terry. But truly, everyone attempting to bulk up or shape their physique is at risk.

You'll need to handle your nutrition and exercise with military precision if you're serious about bodybuilding. If you're trying to gain weight (bulking) or lose fat (cutting) 12 weeks out from a competition, your training program will be drastically different. Naturally, neither of these has much space for a Friday night pint.

Let's not get ahead of ourselves; although difficult, this is doable. The good, the bad, and the traditional information regarding natural bodybuilding are provided here for beginners.

Splits for Bodybuilding Training

How many hours of training should you put in on average each week to get larger and more defined? is a question that almost every newbie has. The answer is that it actually depends on how you separate your training.

However, there are other methods to approach them, such as dividing them into upper and lower body workouts or concentrating on push and pull motions. There are also several scheduling options, such as every other day, four days on and three days off, and so on.

Lat raises in The Bodybuilder's Shoulder Workout for Beginners

lateral dumbbell lift

three sets of 12 repetitions

Pick up some dumbbells that are not too heavy for you to lift. With your elbows slightly bent, hold them close to your sides. Stretch your core while bending your elbows as you stand with your feet shoulder-width apart. Keep your elbows where they are as you raise your arms straight out to your sides to shoulder height. After a brief pause at the peak, slowly drop the weights down to the starting position.

the human leg, shoulder, joint, knee, calf, shorts, muscle, standing

ring of resistance 3 sets of 12 repetitions of raising

Hold the resistance band with an underhand grip while standing on it, holding it about shoulder-width apart. Curl the band so that your forearms are in contact with your biceps and it is parallel to your collarbone. Repeat after lowering.

Pulls three sets of 12 repetitions on each of the following: Arm, Leg, Human Leg, Human Body, Shoulder, Elbow, Standing, Wrist, Joint, and Face.

On a cable machine, attach rope handles to the top pulley. Put your flat foot on the ground and bend down to kneel in front of it. Pulling your hands apart and being careful to maintain your upper arms flat, grab the handles and bring them towards your face. Pause, then reverse the movement

The Beginner Bodybuilder's Leg Workout

Strength training, overhead press, and a barbell Physical fitness, shoulder Free weight bar, fitness gear, Standing, joint, arm

3 sets of 12 repetitions of the barbell back squat

Put more space between your feet than shoulder width. With an overhand grip, hold a barbell across your upper back and hug it into your traps. Squat down carefully while keeping your head up, your back straight, and your buns out. Legs bent at 90 degrees, lower yourself until your hips and knees are in line. To push yourself back up quickly, plant your heels firmly on the ground.

standing, shoulder, leg, knee, exercise apparatus, muscle, and weightlifting machine

Trench-rope pushups

three sets of 12 repetitions

A cable station's high pulley should have a rope handle attached to it. Maintaining a tight core, grip the handle while keeping your elbows tucked in at your sides. Bring your hands down until your arms are completely extended, then return to the starting position. You should just move your forearms.

Weights, exercise equipment Weight training, a barbell, and physical fitness, Bench, arm, weightlifting equipment, gym

skull crusher EZ bar

three sets of 12 repetitions

Straighten your arms up in the air while holding the EZ bar in the inside grips. Slowly lower the bar until it is approximately an inch from your forehead while keeping your elbows firmly planted and tucked in. Without locking your elbows, slowly extend your arms back to the beginning position.

various weight training regimens

It's critical to consistently switch up your regimen, says Terry. It will be simpler once your body is used to performing the same thing every week. Your body will adjust (i.e., plateau) to prevent breaking down muscle groups when feasible since it naturally opposes doing so.

It's not necessary to create a new strategy every three weeks. Naturally, increasing weight and adjusting reps are both crucial for advancement, but experimenting with various set designs can surprise your body and keep things fresh. Keep in mind that growing muscle shouldn't seem like work. To help you gain muscle more effectively during bodybuilding training, we've listed eight distinct types of sets below.

1. Direct Sets

The typical exercise set-up involves performing several sets with the same amount of repetitions and weight, followed by a short break. Starting with this style, you should go to the others.

For instance, perform 10 bench press repetitions, then rest.

Drop Sets 2.

Drop sets provide you the option to work out longer

than you would otherwise. Your muscles are forgetting to state "at that weight" while they are screaming "no more." You may exercise for longer by lifting less weight.

For instance, after doing a leg press to failure, drop the weight quickly. With the new weight, the leg press to failure, then gradually lower the weight without stopping. Go on till you can no longer.

Super Set 3.

When two (or more) exercises for opposing muscle groups are performed back-to-back, without a break, the intensity is increased and you may finish more work in less time.

An illustration would be 10 reps of tricep dips and 10 reps of bicep curls. then take a break.

Compound Set 4.

Similar to a superset, with the exception that you work the same muscle area with two (or more) separate exercises.

Example: Ten bench presses, then ten pushups. then take a break.

diet for bodybuilding

Pyramid Set, No. 5

By progressively lowering the reps and raising the weights with each successive repetition, pyramid sets let you gradually increase the intensity of your workout. The opening set also functions as a warm-up.

Dumbbell chest press, as an illustration, increasing the weight until you can perform 15 repetitions, then 12, then 10, then 8, then

6. No intermission.

With rest-pause training, you're effectively dividing your set into some micro sets, which enables you to go beyond your typical point of failure.

Ex: 8 preacher curls with dumbbells to failure, rest, 3 repetitions to failure, rest, 1 rep to failure.

7. Pressured Time

The term "time under tension" (TUT) training describes how long a muscle works throughout the "eccentric" and "concentric" phases of a session. Your TUT is 30 seconds if you finish 10 repetitions in 3 seconds each. As an illustration, if you raise a weight for two seconds, pause for one second at the top, and then drop it for two seconds, you'll record 50 seconds of total time under tension (TUT) for each rep, even if your muscle is only exerting much more effort.

8. Giant Set and Tri-set

Three exercises for the same body part are performed back-to-back with no break in between as a tri-set. A tri-set with additional exercises and sets is known as a big set.

For illustration, perform 10 squats, 10 leg extensions, and 10 lying hamstring curls.

You keep hearing it, but the most crucial thing is to pay attention to your body. Terry states, "I see how I feel on the day. "I will go for the larger lifts if I'm feeling strong if I've had enough calories and rest, but if I'm dieting, in a calorie deficit, or exhausted, then I'll focus on technique and volume."

And what workouts should be avoided? He cautions against ego-lifting, no matter how tempting it may seem. Testing your 1RM may be cool-looking, but it's not a good approach to developing strength; rather, it's a surefire way to get hurt.

Chapter 2

What most people don't know about body training
Leg Press 1 of 12
Housers Guru / Getty
I have no idea how to work out or utilize the equipment. Where do I begin?
The gym might be scary for someone who is just starting. I advise employing a personal trainer for a minimum of eight to ten sessions because of this. He or she may instruct you on appropriate workout techniques, breathing patterns, and rep cadences in addition to which muscle regions each piece of equipment targets. A qualified

trainer can also assist you in creating a training regimen that is appropriate for your current level of fitness, your specific objectives, and any ailments or physical restrictions you may have.

Bicep curls, 2 of 12, from Inti St. Clair / Getty

What kind of exercise should I perform to reduce my weight?

You need to combine weight/resistance training with aerobic activity if you want to lose weight. Many people make the mistake of doing excessive cardio and skipping weightlifting because they believe that only stair steppers, treadmills, and stationary cycles can burn fat. This is not the case, however.

While exercise will undoubtedly help you burn more calories, weight training will accelerate your metabolism (making you a fat-burning machine), alter your body's composition, and give you the desired form and features. I advise doing cardio at least four to five days a week, either first thing in the morning or immediately after resistance training, and lifting weights three to four days a week.

Deadlifting 3 of 12

How should I workout if I want to gain muscle and strength?

You'll need a well-crafted weight training regimen that largely makes use of free weights and complex (multi-joint) workouts if you want to gain strength and muscle. Most people find that a four-day per week regimen that follows a two on, one off; two on, two off schedule works pretty well. This gives you three days for relaxation and rehabilitation while enabling you to hammer each muscle group hard once every week (which is when actual growth takes place).

For key muscles like the back, quadriceps, hamstrings, chest, and shoulders, I advise beginning with roughly four movements for three sets each. You'll perform well with just three movements for two to three sets each for smaller groups like the biceps, triceps, traps, abs, forearms, and calves. Work sets of 13 to 15, 10 to 12, and 7 to 9 repetitions after each exercise, with one to three warm-up sets (more are required early in the program.)

4 OF 12 A healthy guy uses technology to monitor his exercise to stick to his resolutions

Getty Images/Letizia Le Fur

How long should I work out in the gym?

This relies on your present level of fitness, the objectives you have set for yourself, and the amount of time you have to dedicate to exercising, similar to the last question. It could be better for some people to plan three one-hour exercises each week, whilst others might find it more practical and advantageous to work out five or six days a week for only 30 minutes each time.

To put it another way, it's advisable to estimate how many hours you'll spend at the gym altogether each week before choosing how to divide that time up. Quality of time, as opposed to mere quantity, is a crucial factor to take into account. A person who is committed and concentrated throughout their training may frequently do considerably more in only 30 minutes someone who spends an hour there but is continually distracted by their phone, chit-chatting with others, and simply observing rather than participating.

Westend61/Getty Images 5 OF 12 Resting

How much sleep do I require?

The body must rest longer between sets of some workouts than others since they are far more physically taxing. For instance, a set of 15 barbell squat repetitions would strain your thighs, glutes, and lower back while also making you breathe heavily. You could discover that it takes you three to four minutes to get ready to go on to the next set. On the other hand, it could only take 45 to 60 seconds to recover after executing 15 dumbbell side laterals.

What your main objective is and how weight training can help you achieve it are other factors to take into account. A person working out to bulk up significantly in size and strength will want to take longer breaks in between sets in order to be able to lift the most weight for the most repetitions. Even if the weights are less, it is vital to keep heart rate raised and move fast from set to set if you want to burn body fat and improve endurance.

12 Supplements, 6 OF

David Sacha / Getty

Should I begin taking supplements?

Implementing an educated and effective training routine and a healthy and balanced eating plan should be the major emphasis of your initial health and fitness journey. Anyone who advises you to start using various sports supplements right away is either uninformed or out to make money (well, most of them). It's fine to consider adding supplements to the mix after spending eight to twelve weeks in the gym, exercising hard and regularly while carefully maintaining a healthy diet.

Post-workout Protein: 7 of 12

Is there truly a 30- to 60-minute gap after exercise when one should eat protein? Why?

The body enters a unique metabolic state where protein and carbs are partitioned toward muscles and away from fat cells within the first hour of an intense weight training session. This is because insulin sensitivity is at an all-time high at this time, making it exceedingly easy for amino acids and carbohydrates to enter, digest, and be stored in injured muscle cells. You'll get far greater benefits over time than if you consume your post-workout meal outside of this anabolic window since repair, healing, and recuperation can begin right away.

8 OF 12 Training Out of Shape Getty/Digital Vision

I'm in terrible shape. Is there anything I shouldn't do that is risky?

Even while it's probably safe for you to start a mild exercise regimen, it would be ideal for you to speak with your doctor before even entering a gym, preferably under the supervision of a knowledgeable and experienced personal trainer. Especially when you are taking efforts to enhance your health and wellness, getting the all-clear from your doctor will provide you peace of mind and prevent you from inadvertently causing yourself pain, illness, or accident. Don't be discouraged; simply consult your doctor to obtain a physical and develop a plan of action first.

Hiking Jordan Siemens 9/12

Do you have any suggestions for fitness endeavors or other exercise?

Definitely, sure. Outdoor activities are fantastic for your physical health, but they've also been shown to benefit your mental health. Depression is a common reason why individuals struggle to lose weight. When it comes to getting in your cardiovascular workout, these kinds of activities are particularly helpful. Walking on a treadmill every session is significantly less pleasurable than hiking, dancing, biking, running up and down stairs, or swimming.

Body Fat Calipers, 10 OF 12

IAN SPL/HOOTON / Getty

How can I tell whether my training is effective? What performance indicators ought I to monitor?

When beginning any type of physical fitness program, it is crucial to carefully monitor your progress. Every two to four weeks, if you can, you should see a coach or trainer to have your weight, body fat percentage, and total measurements taken. If you want to go further and control general health indicators like total cholesterol, the ratio of LDL to HDL, triglycerides, and blood pressure, you may do so by getting routine blood tests via your primary care provider.

Unexpectedly, experiencing how your clothing fit is a really excellent sign of success. Naturally, if your shirts are fitting closer through the back, chest, and arms, you know you are on the right track if you want to develop bigger and more muscular. The scale is not necessarily a reliable indicator of how well your program is working because it is highly easy for people, particularly women, to lose multiple sizes without dropping any weight. Always keep in mind that while fat takes up a lot more space, muscle weighs more.

Gym Plateau 11 OF 12 Martin-dm / Getty

What should I do if I reach a plateau?

When development stalls, it's essential to thoroughly review your entire program and decide what adjustments are necessary to resurrect it. Sometimes the solution is as simple as putting in more effort or adjusting your diet by adding or removing calories (depending on the goal). Other times, you have to question whether you are really giving everything you have every workout. Simply turning up won't do the trick; you'll need to pay attention, concentrate, and give each set and rep everything you've got.

Another explanation is that you need a change since your body and mind have grown accustomed to the workouts and cardio you have been performing. Try adjusting the rest period between sets, utilizing a different cardio machine, increasing or decreasing the resistance, or modifying some of your weight training routines.

Tire Flip 12 OF 12 BJI/Blue Jean Images/Getty

I'm having a lot of trouble sticking with it.

The hardest of all the questions to answer could be this one. It need internal motivation and willpower to push oneself day after day. It's up to you to make the journey, even if others close to you provide their support (and you should question anybody who doesn't). You are the one who needs to forgo the cheat meals, abstain from alcohol, lift weights, and work out on the stepper, bike, and treadmill.

Chapter 3

Myth 1: Muscle tissue turns into belly fat if it isn't utilized.
Muscle does not turn into fat while it is inactive; rather, if you are losing muscle, you are probably leading a lifestyle that will also result in the buildup of fat. GSO Pictures/Getty Pictures
It's true that muscles will start to shrink if you stop utilizing them, says Curtis Christopherson, certified personal trainer and CEO of Innovative Fitness.
And since you aren't using those extra calories as fuel, they will probably be stored as body fat if you continue eating

the same number of calories as you did while you were lifting weights.

Myth 2: Lifting weights early thing in the morning helps you get more muscle.

Regardless matter what time of day you work out, the routine that you follow the most religiously will be the one that will help you attain your objectives.

What the research says: A small 2016 study found that men who trained for strength and endurance in the evening compared to the morning had greater increases in muscle mass.

Myth 3: Before working out your muscles, you should stretch.

Instead of static stretching, concentrate on active warm-ups. Images from Yagi Studio/Getty

The American College of Sports Medicine (ACSM) states that "static stretches" kept in place, such as reaching for your toes, have not been shown to increase performance when it comes to stretching before an exercise.

A dynamic warm-up, such as running or jumping jacks, followed by lunges, leg swings, and arm circles is what the ACSM advises practicing in place. This will increase your heart rate, promote blood flow, and allow for a complete range of motion. According to the ACSM, these kinds of motions may improve your overall performance while lowering your chance of injury.

Myth 4: Fat weighs more than muscle.

scales

A pound of fat weighs the same as a pound of muscle. Stillwell/Getty Pictures

A pound of muscle and fat would weigh the same if they were placed on a scale, and according to Garcia, the same is true of your body.

Muscle is more compact than fat, which means it takes up less space in the body. Because of this, two persons with the same weight might seem significantly differently depending on their body composition, or the ratio of muscle to fat.

Myth number five: Lifting weights makes women bulky.

It's less common for women to get bulky from lifting since they naturally have less testosterone, which is necessary for developing large muscles. Getty Pictures

According to research, testosterone has a significant impact in your ability to gain muscle, and women don't make nearly as much testosterone as men do.

Given that testosterone levels in males are typically around ten times greater than in women, it would be very difficult for a woman to seem "bulky," even with regular strength training with heavy weights.

Chapter 4

See the top 6 laws of muscle growth that you must abide by and have in mind as you embark on your fitness path.

Law #1: Workout five days each week.

When it comes to gaining muscle, four to five days per week of training is thought to be the perfect amount. Since it's a lengthy procedure, you should aim for five days, but if time is an issue or you have another problem, attempt to train for at least four days in a row.

Additionally, remember to give yourself a day off in between training sessions and refrain from exercising, for example, three days in a row. This is crucial because your muscles need time to recuperate, and if you don't allow them some downtime, you'll overload your joints and risk injuring your muscles.

Law #2: Allow 2-3 minutes to rest in between exercises

You can be tempted to work out continuously without stopping to rest when growing muscles. You must, however, rest for two to three minutes in between each exercise. This is crucial because you need to give your muscles rest to prevent weariness from activity.

After all, if you overwork your muscles over an extended period, they might get uncomfortable and tired.

Law #3: Ensure That You Have the Correct Form

Fitness jargon describes the form as a specific manner to carry out an activity to prevent injury, build strength, and provide better outcomes. Making sure you have excellent form is one of the most crucial rules of muscle growth since it will help you exercise more effectively and reduce unnecessary movement.

Law #4: Adhere To A Plan

Exercise variety is important since it helps provide a novel stimulus, which eventually results in greater and faster improvement.

With a selection of workouts that focus on the various muscles in your body, design an effective muscle-building regimen. When exercising the biceps, for instance, you might pick movements that provide greater stress on your inner and/or outer biceps to ensure that both get enough work.

Use compound lifts and movements, per Law #5. First

In the gym, you must avoid injuries if you want to make long-term growth. An injury might abruptly stop your development, forcing you to start again from scratch.

Therefore, starting with compound lifts and motions is the best course of action in this situation.

In essence, compound workouts work for many muscular groups at once. A popular illustration of this is a squat, which simultaneously works your glutes, quadriceps, and calves. Because they engage numerous muscles at once, compound exercises are excellent for beginners because they reduce stress on a single muscle.

Law # 6 – Take Proper Nutrition and Sleep for Recovery

No matter how hard you work out in the gym, if you don't get enough sleep and the right nutrition, you aren't likely to build muscle successfully. A core requirement for building muscle is proper nutrition in the form of fats, proteins, and good carbohydrates.

Alongside this, you need a good night's sleep to ensure muscle recovery because your body repairs itself and grows while you're sleeping.

Follow these laws of muscle building during your fitness regime, and you will be able to achieve that body you've always dreamed of!

www.ingramcontent.com/pod-product-compliance
Lightning Source LLC
LaVergne TN
LVHW052114160826
845678LV00015B/3549

* 9 7 9 8 3 5 1 8 4 5 1 8 0 *